YOUR GUIDE TO
Physical Activity and
Your Heart

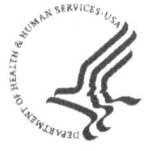
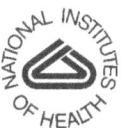
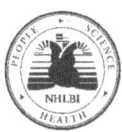

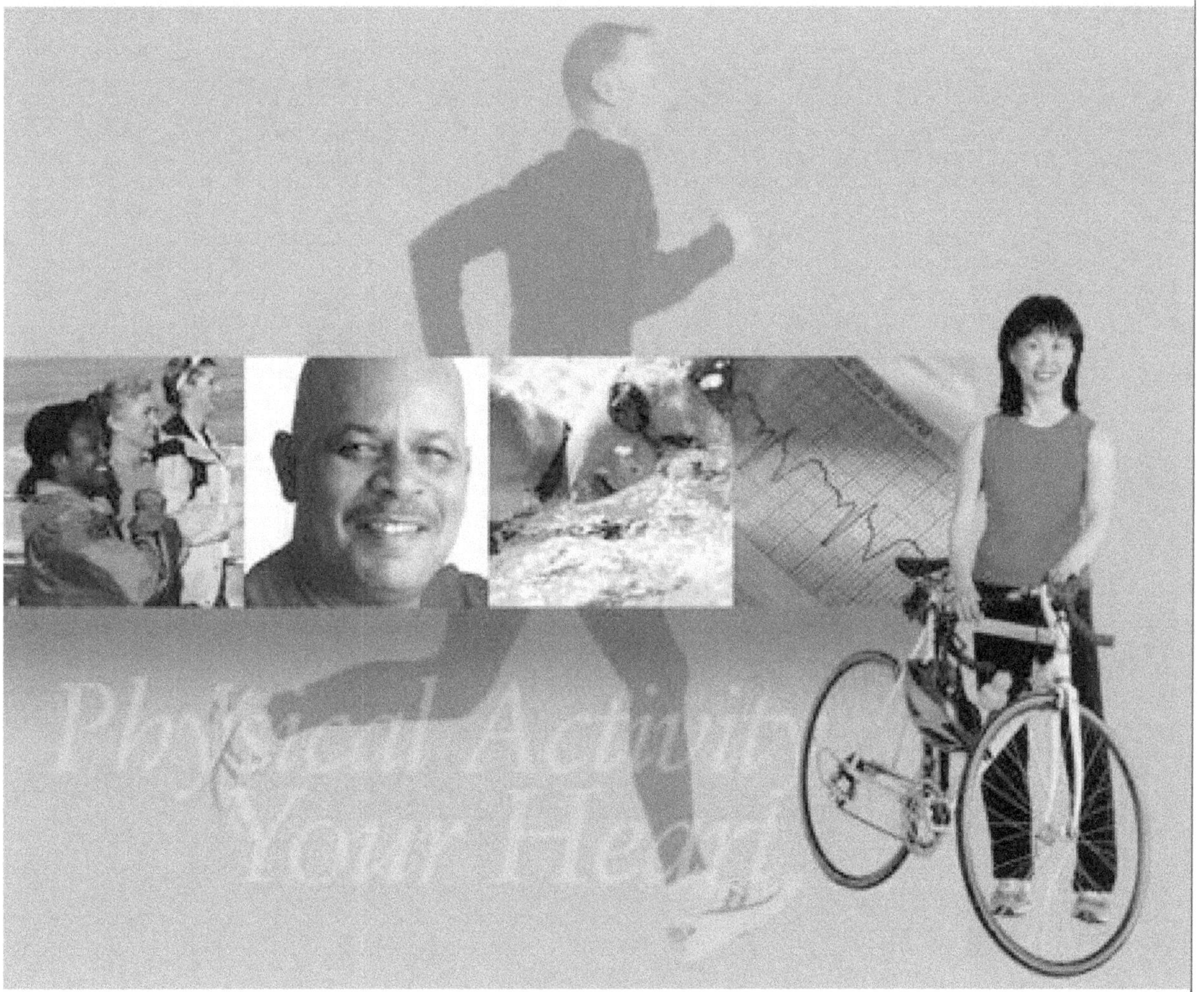

U.S. DEPARTMENT OF HEALTH AND HUMAN SERVICES
National Institutes of Health
National Heart, Lung, and Blood Institute

NIH Publication No. 06-5714
June 2006

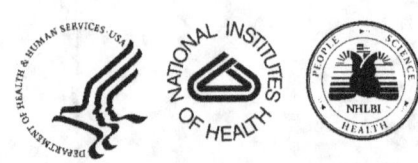

U.S. DEPARTMENT OF HEALTH AND HUMAN SERVICES
National Institutes of Health
National Heart, Lung, and Blood Institute

Contents

On the Move

Chances are, you already know that physical activity is good for you. "Sure," you may say. "When I get out and move around, I know it helps me to feel and look better." But you may not realize just how important regular physical activity is to your health.

According to the U.S. Surgeon General's Report on Physical Activity and Health, **inactive people are nearly twice as likely to develop heart disease as those who are more active.** This is true even if you have no other conditions or habits that increase your risk for heart disease. Lack of physical activity also leads to more visits to the doctor, more hospitalizations, and more use of medicines for a variety of illnesses.

The good news is that physical activity can protect your heart in a number of important ways. Moreover, to get benefits, you don't have to run a marathon. Regular activity—something as simple as a brisk, 30-minute walk each day—can help you to reduce your risk of heart disease.

This booklet will help you to understand the impact of physical activity on your heart, as well as the power of regular activity to help keep you healthy overall. It will also offer plenty of ideas on starting a physical activity program that will be both healthful and enjoyable. Just as important, you'll get tips for keeping up with the activity or activities you choose, since staying active over time is important to long-term health. So use this booklet often for information, ideas, and to keep you motivated. When to start getting fit? There's no time like today.

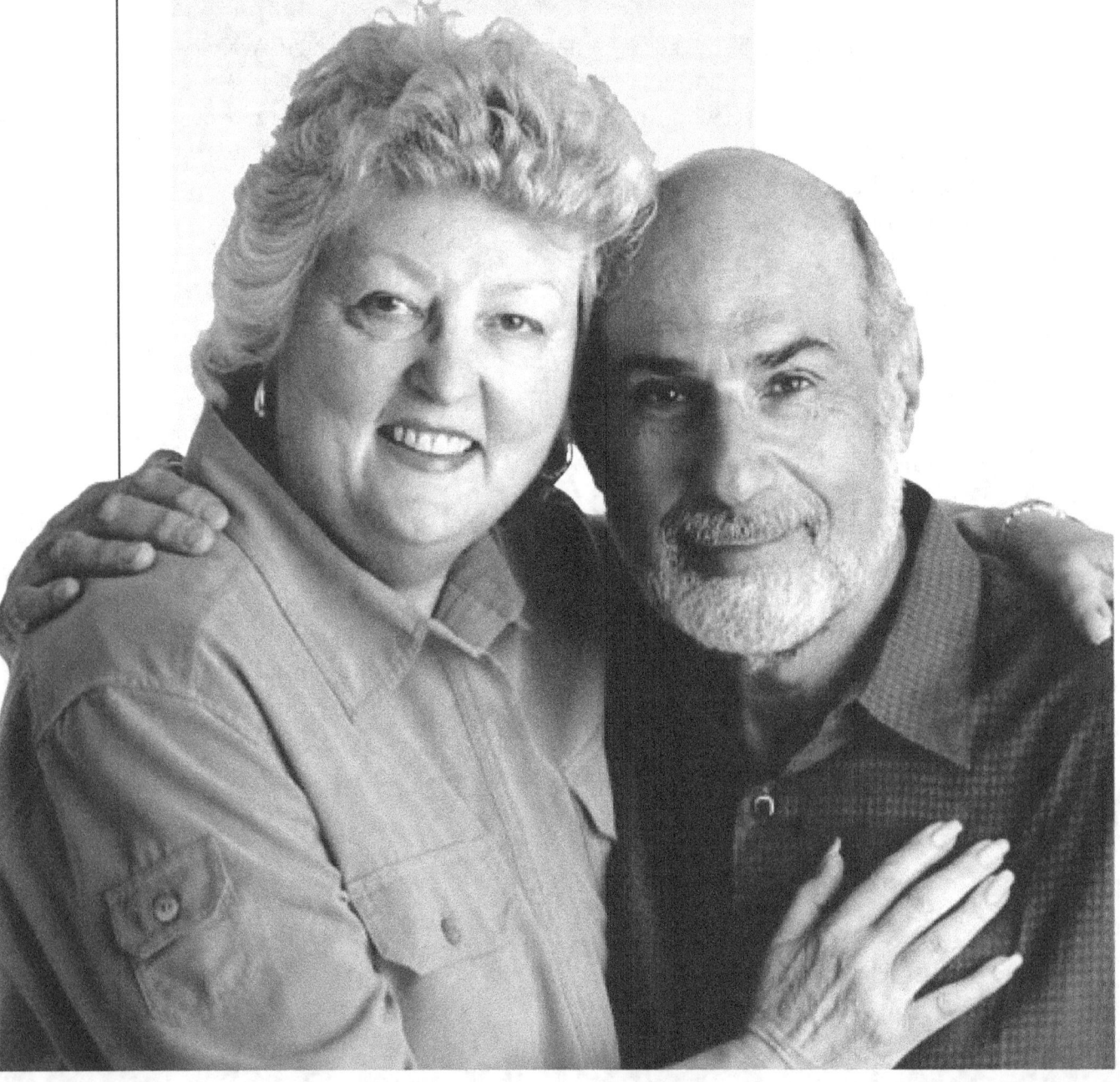

ALAN AND LILA LETOW

"Exercise and taking good care of ourselves are important parts of our life plan. Lila and I exercise regularly and look to not only cardiovascular and strength building exercises, but also to improving our muscle flexibility and range of motion. Hopefully, this should keep us fit for the years ahead."

Physical Activity and Your Health

If you currently get regular physical activity, congratulations! But if you're not yet getting all the activity you need, you have lots of company. According to the Centers for Disease Control and Prevention (CDC), 60 percent of Americans are not meeting the recommended levels of physical activity. Fully 16 percent of Americans are not active at all. Overall, women tend to be less active than men, and older people are less likely to get regular physical activity than younger individuals.

What does it mean to get "regular physical activity?" To reduce the risk of heart disease, adults need only do about 30 minutes of moderate activity on most, and preferably all, days of the week. This level of activity can also lower your chances of having a stroke, colon cancer, high blood pressure, diabetes, and other medical problems.

If you're also trying to manage your weight and prevent gradual, unhealthy weight gain, try to get 60 minutes of moderate- to vigorous-intensity activity on most days of the week. At the same time, watch your calories. Take in only enough calories to maintain your weight. Those who are trying to keep weight off should aim a bit higher: Try to get 60–90 minutes of moderate-intensity activity daily, without taking in extra calories. Later in the book, you'll find out more about the types of activities that you can easily fit into your routine, as well as ways to break up your activity time into manageable segments.

If you're not as active as you might be, take a moment to consider why. Maybe you're just in the habit of traveling by car or bus, even when you're not going far. In your free time, perhaps it's tempting to sit down in front of the TV or computer rather than do something more vigorous. It's easy to get busy or tired and decide that it's just simpler to put off that brisk walk or bike ride. But when you think about the serious problems that physical inactivity can create for your health—and the enormous rewards of getting regular activity—

you may want to reconsider. Let's start with the ways that physical activity affects your heart.

Physical Activity: The Heart Connection

It's worth repeating: Physical inactivity greatly increases your risk of developing heart disease. Heart disease occurs when the arteries that supply blood to the heart muscle become hardened and narrowed, due to a buildup of plaque on the arteries' inner walls. Plaque is the accumulation of fat, cholesterol, and other substances. As plaque continues to build up in the arteries, blood flow to the heart is reduced.

Heart disease can lead to a heart attack. A heart attack happens when a cholesterol-rich plaque bursts and releases its contents into the bloodstream. This causes a blood clot to form over the plaque, totally blocking blood flow through the artery and preventing vital oxygen and nutrients from getting to the heart. A heart attack can cause permanent damage to the heart muscle.

Some people aren't too concerned about heart disease because they think it can be cured with surgery. This is a myth. Heart disease is a lifelong condition. It's true that certain procedures can help blood and oxygen flow more easily to the heart. But the arteries remain damaged, which means you are still more likely to have a heart attack. What's more, the condition of your blood vessels will steadily worsen unless you make changes in your daily habits and control other factors that increase risk.

Heart disease is a serious disease—and too often, a fatal one. It is the number one killer of Americans, with 500,000 people in the United States dying of heart disease each year. Many others with heart problems become permanently disabled. That's why it's so vital to take action to prevent this disease. Getting regular physical activity should be part of everyone's heart disease prevention program.

Heart Disease Risk Factors

Risk factors are conditions or habits that make a person more likely to develop a disease. They can also increase the chances that an existing disease will get worse. Certain risk factors for heart disease, such as getting older or having a family history of early heart disease, can't be changed. But **physical inactivity is a major risk factor for heart disease that you have control over.** You can make a decision to get regular physical activity, and this booklet can help you create a workable, enjoyable program that will help you protect your heart.

Other major risk factors for heart disease that you can change are smoking, high blood pressure, high blood cholesterol, overweight, and diabetes. (See the box, "You Have Control," on page 6.) Every risk factor counts. Research shows that each individual risk factor greatly increases the chances of developing heart disease and having a heart attack. A damaged heart can damage your life, by interfering with enjoyable activities and even keeping you from doing simple things, such as taking a walk or climbing steps.

But it's important to know that you have a lot of power to protect your heart health. (See the box, "Eight Tips for Heart Health," on page 7.) Getting regular physical activity is an especially important part of your healthy heart program, because physical activity both directly reduces your heart disease risk *and* reduces your chances of developing other risk factors for heart disease. For example, regular physical activity may reduce LDL (bad) cholesterol, increase HDL (good) cholesterol, and lower high blood pressure. It can also protect your heart by helping to prevent and control diabetes. Finally, physical activity can help you to lose excess weight or stay at your desirable weight, which will also help to lower your risk of

You Have Control

Physical inactivity is one of several major risk factors for heart disease that you can do something about. The others are:

Smoking. People who smoke are up to six times more likely to suffer a heart attack than nonsmokers, and the risk increases with the number of cigarettes smoked each day. Quitting will greatly reduce your risk. Check with local community groups for free or low cost programs designed to help people stop smoking.

High Blood Pressure. Also known as hypertension, high blood pressure increases your risk of heart disease, stroke, kidney disease, and congestive heart failure. Your health care provider can check your blood pressure by means of a simple test using an inflatable arm cuff. Blood pressure often can be entirely controlled by getting regular physical activity, losing excess weight, cutting down on alcohol, and changing eating habits, such as using less salt and other forms of sodium. For some people, medication is also needed.

High Blood Cholesterol. High blood cholesterol can lead to the buildup of plaque in your arteries, which raises the risk of a heart attack. Starting at age 20, everyone should have their cholesterol levels checked by means of a blood test called a "lipoprotein profile." You can lower high blood cholesterol by getting regular physical activity, eating less saturated fat and *trans* fat, and managing your weight. In some cases, medication is also needed.

Overweight. If you are overweight or obese, you are more likely to develop heart disease even if you have no other risk factors. Ask your doctor to help you determine whether you need to lose weight for your health. The good news: Losing just 5 10 percent of your current weight will help to lower your risk of heart disease and many other medical disorders.

Diabetes greatly increases your risk for heart disease, stroke, and other serious diseases. Ask your doctor whether you should be tested for it. Many people at high risk for diabetes can prevent or delay the disease by reducing calories as part of a healthy eating plan, and by becoming more physically active. If you already have diabetes, work closely with your doctor to manage it.

Eight Tips for Heart Health

- Become and stay physically active.
- Balance your calorie intake with the calories you burn in physical activity.
- Lose weight if you're overweight.
- If you smoke, stop. Avoid other people's smoke if you can.
- Control high blood pressure.
- Control high blood cholesterol.
- Control diabetes.
- Choose foods low in saturated fat, *trans* fat, cholesterol, sugar, and salt. Enjoy more fruits, vegetables, and whole grains.

heart disease.

Physical Activity: The Calorie Connection

One way that regular physical activity protects against heart disease is by burning extra calories, which helps you to lose excess weight or stay at your desirable weight. To understand how physical activity affects calories, it is helpful to consider the concept of "energy balance." Energy balance is the amount of calories you take in relative to the amount of calories you burn. Per week, you need to burn off about 3,500 more calories than you take in to lose 1 pound. If you need to lose weight for your health, regular physical activity can help you through one of two approaches.

First, you can choose to eat your usual amount of calories, but be more active. For example, a 200-pound person who keeps on eating the same amount of calories, but begins to walk briskly each day for 1½ miles, will lose about 14 pounds in 1 year. Staying active will also help to keep the weight off.

Second, you can eat fewer calories and be more active. This is the best way to lose weight, since you're more likely to be successful by combining a healthful, lower-calorie diet with physical activity. For example, a 200-pound person who consumes 250 fewer calories per day, and begins to walk briskly each day for 1½ miles, will lose about 40 pounds in 1 year.

Most of the energy you burn each day—about three quarters of it—

goes to activities that your body automatically engages in for survival, such as breathing, sleeping, and digesting food. The part of your energy output that *you* control is daily physical activity. Any activity you take part in beyond your body's automatic activities will burn extra calories. Even seated activities, such as using the computer or watching TV, will burn calories—but only a very small number. That's why it's important to make time each day for moderate-to-vigorous physical activity.

The Benefits Keep Coming

It is hard to imagine a single practice with more health benefits than regular physical activity. In addition to protecting your heart in numerous ways, staying active:

▪ May help to prevent cancers of the breast, uterus, and colon.

▪ Strengthens your lungs and helps them to work more efficiently.

▪ Tones and strengthens your muscles.

▪ Builds stamina.

▪ Keeps your joints in good condition.

▪ Improves balance.

▪ May slow bone loss.

Regular physical activity can also boost the way you feel. It may:

▪ Give you more energy.

▪ Help you to relax and cope better with stress.

▪ Build confidence.

▪ Allow you to fall asleep more quickly and sleep more soundly.

▪ Help you to beat the blues.

▪ Provide an enjoyable way to share time with friends or family.

Go for the Burn!

Some physical activities burn more calories than others. Below are the average number of calories a 154 pound person will burn, per hour, for a variety of activities. (A lighter person will burn fewer calories; a heavier person will burn more.) As you can see, vigorous intensity activities burn more calories than moderate intensity activities.

Moderate Physical Activity	Calories Burned per Hour
Hiking	370
Light gardening/yard work	330
Dancing	330
Golf (walking and carrying clubs)	330
Bicycling (less than 10 mph)	290
Walking (3.5 mph)	280
Weight lifting (light workout)	220
Stretching	180

Vigorous Physical Activity	Calories Burned per Hour
Running/jogging	590
Bicycling (more than 10 mph)	590
Swimming (slow freestyle laps)	510
Aerobics	480
Walking (4.5 mph)	460
Heavy yard work (chopping wood, for example)	440
Weight lifting (vigorous workout)	440
Basketball (vigorous)	440

Source: Adapted from the 2005 Dietary Guidelines Advisory Committee Report

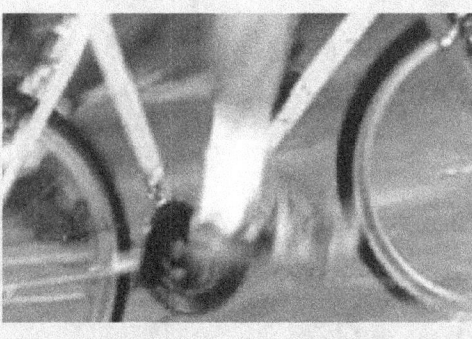

LILY KRAMER

"I think exercise is extremely important. Whenever I feel stressed out, I go to the gym and work out. I come out of there feeling much better."

Great Moves

Given the numerous benefits of regular physical activity, you may be ready to get in motion! But first, it's important to know how activities differ from one another and how each form of movement uniquely contributes to your health. Three types of activity are important for a complete physical activity program: aerobic activity, resistance training, and flexibility exercises. Let's take a brief look at each one.

Types of Physical Activity

Aerobic activity is any physical activity that uses large muscle groups and causes your body to use more oxygen than it would while resting. This booklet focuses mainly on aerobic activity because it is the type of movement that most benefits the heart. Examples of aerobic activity are brisk walking, jogging, and bicycling.

Resistance training—also called strength training—can firm, strengthen, and tone your muscles, as well as improve bone strength, balance, and coordination. Examples of strength moves are pushups, lunges, and bicep curls using dumbbells.

Flexibility exercises stretch and lengthen your muscles. These activities help to improve joint flexibility and keep muscles limber, thereby preventing injury. An example of a stretching move is sitting cross-legged on the floor and gently pushing down on the tops of your legs to stretch the inner thigh muscles.

Working Together for Health

While aerobic activities benefit the heart most, all three types of movement are vital components of a physical activity program. They also work together in important ways. For example, resistance exercises can help you achieve the muscle strength, balance, and coordination to do your aerobic activities more successfully. Meanwhile, flexibility training will help you to move your muscles and joints more easily and prevent injury as you engage in aerobic activities. Many activities that promote flexibility and strength are also relaxing and fun. (See the box, "Three Moves for Health," on page 13.) Below is a sample schedule for a well-rounded activity program.

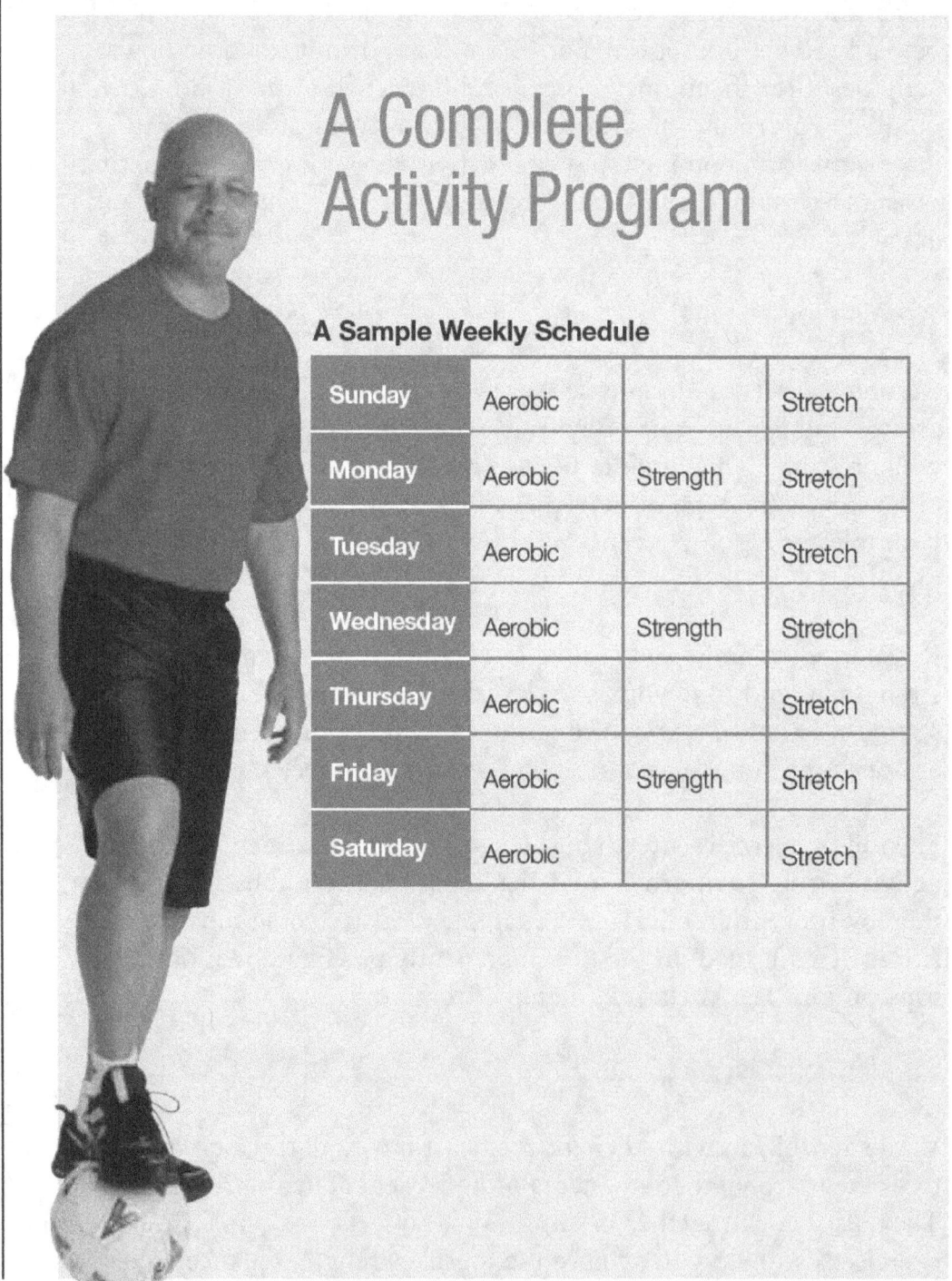

A Complete Activity Program

A Sample Weekly Schedule

Sunday	Aerobic		Stretch
Monday	Aerobic	Strength	Stretch
Tuesday	Aerobic		Stretch
Wednesday	Aerobic	Strength	Stretch
Thursday	Aerobic		Stretch
Friday	Aerobic	Strength	Stretch
Saturday	Aerobic		Stretch

Three Moves for Health

While not usually aerobic, the activities below offer numerous health benefits and are enjoyable ways to get and stay in shape. All are offered at many YMCAs, community or recreation centers, and gyms.

- **Yoga** is a system of physical postures, stretching, and breathing techniques that can improve flexibility, balance, muscle strength, and relaxation. Many styles are available, ranging from slow and gentle to athletic and vigorous. A recent study found that regular yoga practice may help to minimize weight gain in middle age.

- **Tai chi** is an ancient Chinese practice based on shifting body weight through a series of slow movements that flow rhythmically together into one graceful gesture. This gentle, calming practice can help to improve flexibility and balance, and it gradually builds muscle strength.

- **Pilates** is a body conditioning routine that seeks to strengthen the body's "core" (torso), usually through a series of mat exercises. Another Pilates method uses special exercise machines, available at some health clubs. The practice can strengthen and tone muscles as well as increase flexibility.

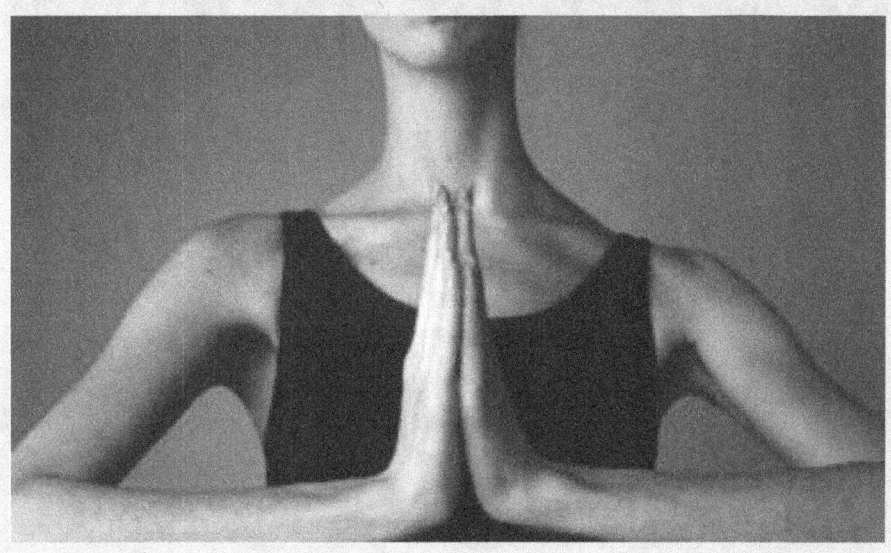

Intensity Levels

Generally, the more vigorously you engage in an activity, and the more time you spend doing it, the more health benefits you will receive. The vigorous activities listed in the left column of the box, "Choosing Your Moves," page 15, are especially helpful for conditioning your heart and lungs, and these activities also burn more calories than those that are less vigorous. However, moderate-intensity activities can also be excellent fitness choices. When done briskly for 30 minutes or longer on most days of the week, the moderate-intensity activities listed in the column on the right side of the box can help to condition your heart and lungs and reduce your risk of heart disease.

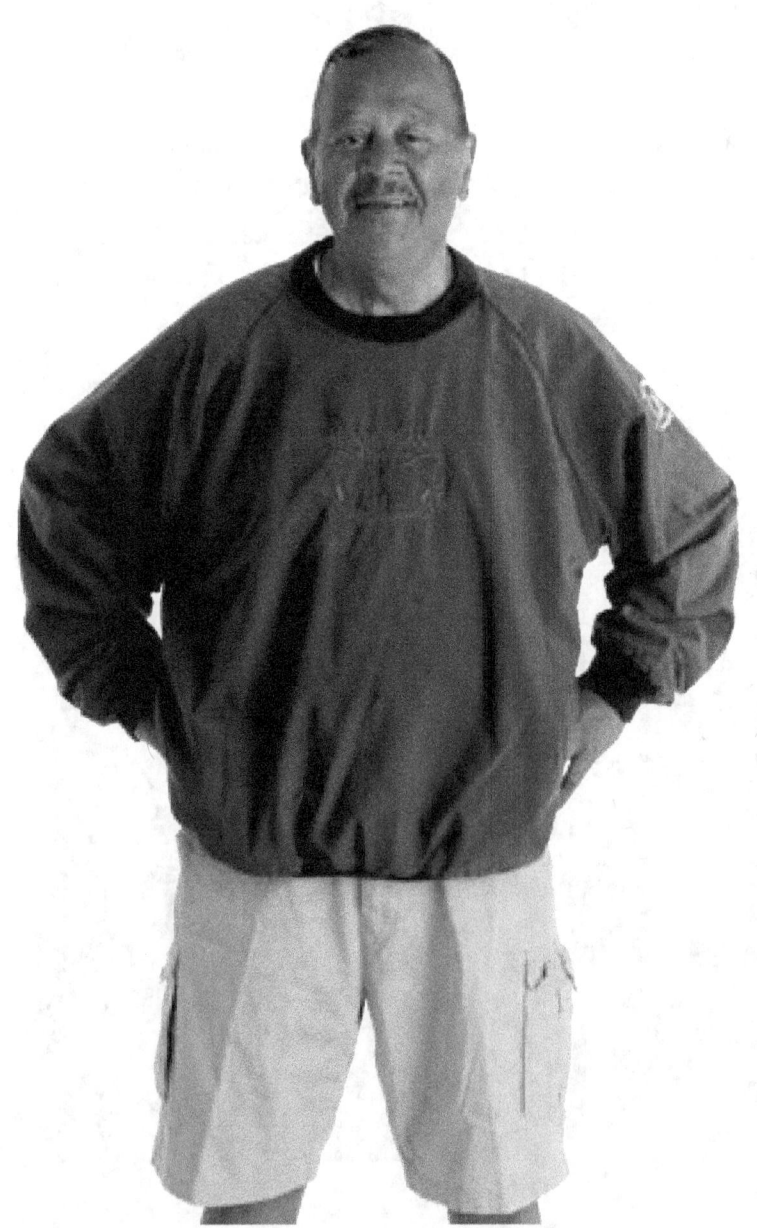

Choosing Your Moves

Vigorous activity	Moderate activity
Aerobic dancing	Bicycling (less than 10 mph)
Basketball	Downhill skiing
Bicycling (more than 10 mph)	Dancing
Cross country skiing	Gardening
Hiking (uphill)	Golf (on foot)
Ice hockey/field hockey	Hiking (flat ground)
Jogging/running (at least 5 mph)	Horseback riding
Jumping rope	Roller skating/ice skating
Soccer	Softball
Stair climbing	Swimming
Tennis (singles)	Tennis (doubles)
Walking briskly (4.5 mph)	Walking moderately (3.5 mph)
Weight lifting (vigorous effort)	Weight lifting (moderate effort)
Yard work (heavy)	Yard work (light)

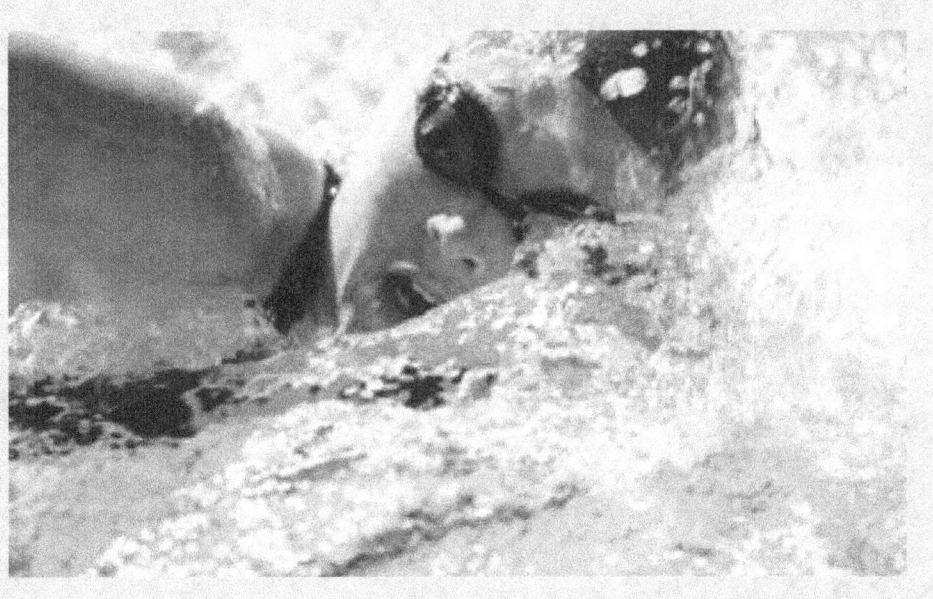

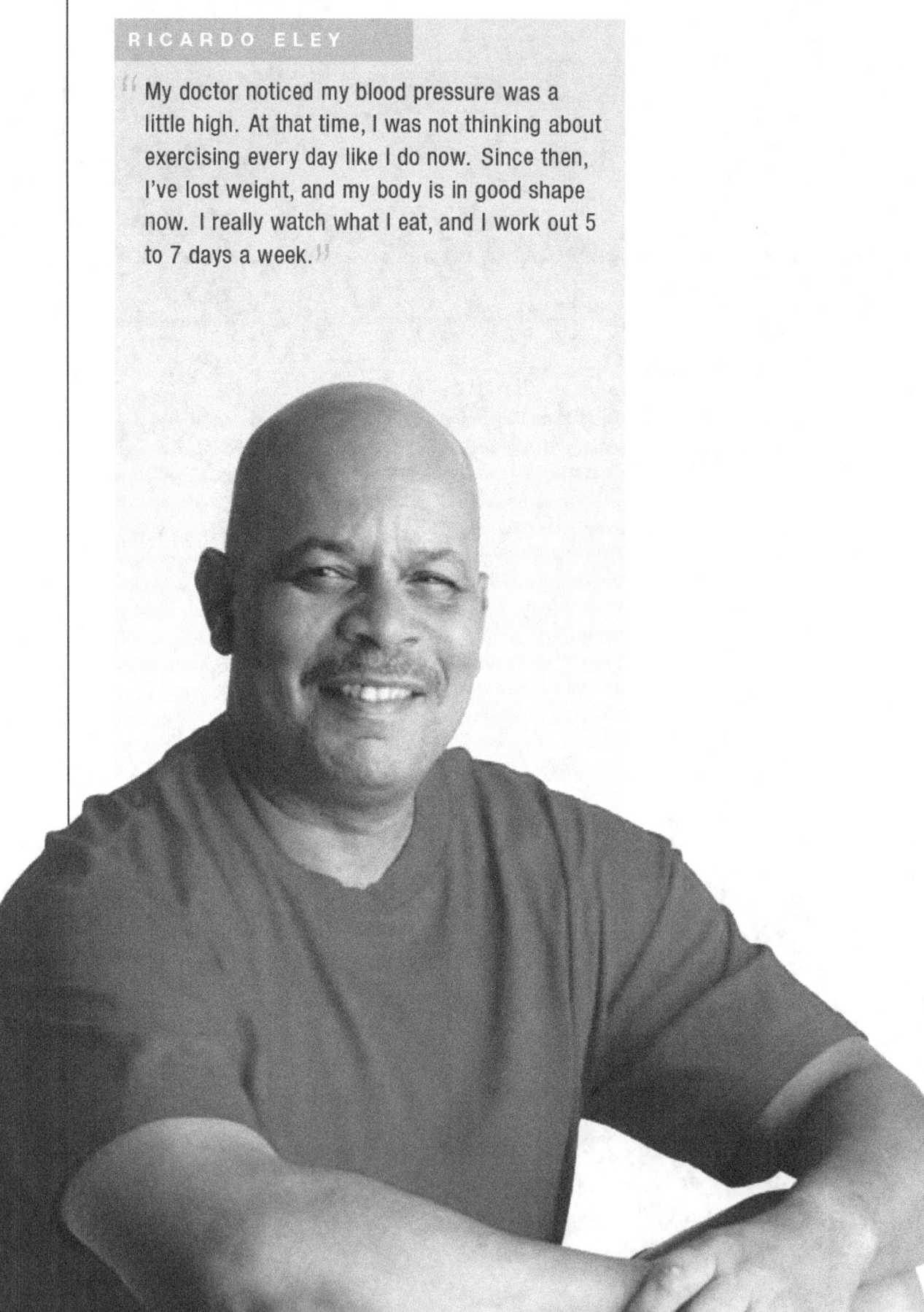

RICARDO ELEY

"My doctor noticed my blood pressure was a little high. At that time, I was not thinking about exercising every day like I do now. Since then, I've lost weight, and my body is in good shape now. I really watch what I eat, and I work out 5 to 7 days a week."

Getting in Motion

Ready to get moving? If so, getting health benefits from regular activity may be easier than you think. As discussed at the start of this book, about 30 minutes of moderate-intensity physical activity on most—and preferably all—days of the week will help you to reduce the risk of heart disease. If you can gradually work up to more time being active, you'll get even more benefits.

Brisk walking is a simple, enjoyable way to help keep your heart healthy. One study showed that regular, brisk walking reduced the risk of heart attack by the same amount as more vigorous exercise, such as jogging. Keep in mind, too, that you can break up any activity into shorter periods of at least 10 minutes each. For example, if you want to total 30 minutes of activity per day, you could spend 10 minutes walking on your lunch break, another 10 minutes raking leaves in the backyard, and another 10 minutes lifting weights. See pages 27–29 for sample walking and jogging programs.

Exploding the Myths

Even when you know physical activity is good for you, it's easy to keep dragging your feet—literally. We all have reasons to stay inactive, but sometimes those reasons are based more on myth than reality. Here are some of the most common myths about physical activity and ways to replace them with a more realistic, can-do spirit.

Myth 1: "Physical activity takes too much time."

Physical activity does take some time, but there are ways to make it manageable. If you don't have 30 minutes in your daily schedule for an activity break, try to find three 10-minute periods. If you're aiming for 60 minutes daily—a good goal if you're trying to avoid weight gain—perhaps you can carve out some "fitness time" early in the day, before your schedule gets too busy. Another idea is to combine physical activity with a task that's already part of your daily routine, such as walking the dog or doing yard chores.

Myth 2: "Getting in shape makes you tired."

Once you begin regular physical activity, you're likely to have even more energy than before. As you progress, daily tasks will seem easier. Regular, moderate-to-brisk physical activity can also help you to reduce fatigue and manage stress.

Myth 3: "The older you are, the less physical activity you need."

Most people become less physically active as they age, but keeping fit is important throughout life. Regular physical activity increases older people's ability to perform routine daily tasks and to stay independent longer. No matter what your age, you can find a physical activity program that is tailored to your particular fitness level and needs.

Myth 4: "Taking medication interferes with physical activity."

In most cases, this is not true. In fact, becoming more active may lessen your need for certain medicines, such as high blood pressure drugs. However, before beginning a physical activity program, be sure to inform your doctor about both prescription and over-the-counter medications you are taking, so that your health can be properly monitored.

Myth 5: "You have to be athletic to exercise."

Most physical activities don't require any special athletic skills. In fact, many people who have bad memories of difficult school sports have discovered a whole world of enjoyable, healthful activities that involve no special talent or training. A perfect example is brisk walking—a superb, heart healthy activity. Others include bicycling, gardening, or yard work, as long as they're done at a brisk pace. Just do more of the activities you already like and already know how to do. It's that simple.

Taking Precautions

Some people should get medical advice before starting, or significantly increasing, physical activity. Check with your doctor first if you:

- Are over 50 years old and not used to moderately energetic activity.

- Currently have a heart condition, have developed chest pain within the last month, or have had a heart attack. (Also see the section, "After a Heart Attack.")

- Have a parent or sibling who developed heart disease at an early age.

- Have any other chronic health problem or risk factors for a chronic disease.

- Tend to easily lose your balance or become dizzy.

- Feel extremely breathless after mild exertion.

- Are on any type of medication.

After a Heart Attack

Following a heart attack, some people are afraid to be physically active. But it's important to know that regular, moderate physical activity can help reduce your risk of having another heart attack and actually improve your chances of survival. Being active can also help you to more easily perform everyday tasks and to do so without chest pain or shortness of breath.

If you've had a heart attack, it's important to consult your doctor to be sure you're following a safe and effective physical activity program. Your doctor's guidance can help prevent heart pain and/or further damage from too much exertion. Ask about getting involved in cardiac rehabilitation, which is a total program for heart health that includes exercise training, education, and counseling to help you return to an active life.

Choosing the Right Activity

The key to a successful fitness program is choosing an activity or activities that will work well for you. Here are some questions to ask yourself to help you find a good "movement match."

1. How physically fit are you?

If you've been inactive for a while, you may want to start with walking, biking, or swimming at a comfortable pace. Beginning with less strenuous activities will allow you to become gradually more fit without straining your body. If you're not sure how physically fit you are, you may want to visit a qualified exercise professional at a local health club or recreation center to receive a fitness assessment. A brief series of physical tests can estimate your current aerobic capacity, strength, and flexibility, as well as measuring your height, weight, and blood pressure. This information can give you a good picture of the shape you're in and allow you to choose activities and goals that are right for you.

2. What kinds of benefits do you want from physical activity?

Aerobic activity benefits the heart and lungs most. Resistance exercises can provide some aerobic conditioning, while also strengthening and toning muscles. Stretching exercises help to keep muscles limber, thereby preventing injury during your physical activity. (See "Types of Physical Activity" on page 11 for more on each form of activity.) The most healthful physical activity program includes all three types of movement.

3. Do you prefer to be active on your own, or with others?

Do you lean toward individual activities, such as swimming or weight lifting; two-person activities, such as dancing; or group sports, such as softball or doubles tennis? If you like to be active with others, consider whether you can find a partner or group easily and quickly. If not, choose another activity until you can find a partner. If you prefer do-it-yourself activities, it may be simpler to get started—but a bit more challenging to maintain your momentum. Choosing an activity you truly enjoy will help you to stay with your activity program.

4. Do you prefer to be active outdoors or in your home?

Both have advantages. Outdoor activities offer variety in scenery and weather. Indoor activities offer shelter from bad weather and the convenience of not having to step beyond your front door. Some activities, such as bench stepping or running in place, can be done indoors or outdoors. If your activity can be seriously affected by weather, consider choosing a second, alternate activity that you can do at home or in a gym.

5. Are you looking for an inexpensive way to get in shape?

Many activities are free or nearly so, requiring no equipment or special clothing. For example, brisk walking requires only a comfortable pair of rubber-soled shoes. Many communities offer free or very affordable physical activity options. Check with your local park and recreation department, which may offer a number of low-cost physical activity classes that are enjoyable for the entire family.

6. Would you like to join a gym or work with a fitness professional?

Some people find that regularly going to a health club, and/or working with a fitness trainer, helps them to stay more motivated. Before you purchase a gym membership or sessions with a professional, be sure to shop around and ask questions.

- Check out the certifications and education of the staff to ensure that they are properly qualified. Professional qualifications include a college degree in a health-related field, such as exercise science or physical education. Ideally, staff should hold an exercise certification from a nationally recognized, nonprofit organization, such as the American College of Sports Medicine.

- Ask to speak to a few current clients to find out about the quality, size, and availability of sessions.

- Pay a visit to the facilities to check out the availability and quality of the equipment, the accessibility of parking, and the travel time from your home or office.

BILL KIRWAN

"I realize I'm not as young as I used to be. I began working out doing both weights and cardio work. Over time, the more I exercised, the more I built up and increased the weights, the more I began to see the benefits. It's a stress reliever. I'm the father of two young boys and they are very active in sports, and now I have the ability to do more of that with them."

▪ Find out about all costs in advance. Fees for fitness services can vary greatly, so be sure to do a cost comparison of gyms and fitness professionals in your area.

7. What is the best time of day for you to be active?

Do you feel more like being active in the morning, afternoon, or evening? If you can, schedule your workouts for times when you feel reasonably energetic. Remember that physical activity sessions can be spread out over the day and needn't take more than 10 minutes at a time.

Smart Moves

Once you find a physical activity that's a good match for you, you're ready for action! But be sure to pace yourself. Each session to condition your heart and lungs should include the following:

Warmup (5 minutes). Start your physical activity session at a slow-to-medium pace to give your body a chance to warm up and get ready for more vigorous movement. Gradually increase your pace by the end of the warm-up period. For especially strenuous activities, such as jumping rope or jogging, warm up for up to 10 minutes.

Be active. Slowly increase your physical activity time until you reach your goal of 30 to 60 minutes daily. To condition your heart and lungs, you should engage in your activity in your "target heart rate zone." (See "Tracking Your Target Heart Rate" on page 24.) But don't focus on big goals in the beginning. If you haven't been active in a while, you might start with just 5–10 minutes of activity per day—or whatever amount of time you're comfortable with. Build up gradually. Enjoy yourself.

Cool down (5 minutes). After being active, slow down gradually. For example, if you've been swimming, begin to do your stroke more slowly, or switch to a more leisurely type of stroke. You can also cool down by changing to a less vigorous activity, such as moving from jogging to walking. This process allows your body to relax gradually. Stopping abruptly can cause dizziness.

Stretch. It's best to do stretching exercises after your activity period, to increase muscle and joint flexibility. Below are several stretches you can use after your cool-down period. Each of these moves helps to stretch different parts of your body. Do each stretch slowly and steadily, without bouncing.

- *Calf wall push*. Stand facing a wall, about 1½ feet away from it. Then lean forward and push your hands against the wall, keeping your heels flat. Count to 10 (or to 20 for a longer stretch). Rest. Repeat.

- *Hamstring palm touch*. Stand with your knees slightly bent. Then, bend from the waist and try to touch your palms to the floor. If you can't reach all the way to the floor, just go as far as you can. Count to 10 or 20, then rest. Repeat. If you have lower back problems, do this stretch with your legs crossed.

- *Hamstring toe touch*. Place your right leg level with your hip on a stair, chair, or other steady object. With your other leg slightly bent, lean forward and slowly try to touch your right toe with your right hand. Hold and count to 10 or 20. Repeat with your left hand. Then switch legs and repeat with each hand. Rest. Repeat the entire stretch.

- *Overhead triceps stretch*. Bend your right elbow and use your left arm to bring it up behind your head. You should feel a gentle stretch on the outside of your upper right arm. Hold for 10 to 20 seconds. Repeat with the left elbow behind your head. Rest. Repeat.

- *Standing quadriceps stretch*. Place your left hand on a chair or wall for support, bend your right knee, and reach back with your right hand to grab the top of your right foot. Hold for 10 to 20 seconds. Repeat on the left side. Rest. Repeat.

Tracking Your Target Heart Rate

As you become more physically active, how will you know whether you're improving your heart and lung fitness? The best way is to track your target heart rate during your activity. Your target heart rate is a percentage of your maximum heart rate, which is the fastest

Finding Your Target Heart Rate Zone

Age	Target Heart Rate Zone: 50–75%	Maximum Heart Rate: 100%
20	100 150 beats per min.	200 beats per min.
25	98 146 beats per min.	195 beats per min.
30	95 142 beats per min.	190 beats per min.
35	93 138 beats per min.	185 beats per min.
40	90 135 beats per min.	180 beats per min.
45	88 131 beats per min.	175 beats per min.
50	85 127 beats per min.	170 beats per min.
55	83 123 beats per min.	165 beats per min.
60	80 120 beats per min.	160 beats per min.
65	78 116 beats per min.	155 beats per min.
70	75 113 beats per min.	150 beats per min.

your heart can beat, based on your age. Unless you're in excellent physical condition, any physical activity that boosts your heart rate above 75 percent of your maximum rate is likely to be too strenuous. By the same token, any activity that increases your heart rate to less than 50 percent of your maximum rate gives your heart and lungs too little conditioning.

Getting Into the Zone

The most healthful activity level uses 50–75 percent of your maximum heart rate. This range, called your **target heart rate zone**, is shown above. During the first few months of your activity program, aim to reach 50 percent of your maximum rate. As you get into better shape, you can slowly build up to 75 percent.

Keep in mind that "getting into the zone" doesn't mean pushing yourself to the limit. For example, while walking briskly or jogging, you should be able to keep up a conversation without trouble. If you can't, move a bit more slowly. Overall, a gentle, gradual approach will help you to maximize your gains and minimize your risks. (See "A Sample Walking Program" on page 27 and "A Sample Jogging Program" on page 28.)

What's Your Number?

To find your target heart rate zone, look for the age closest to yours in the table on page 25. For example, if you're 40, your target zone is 90–135 beats per minute. If you're 53, the closest age on the chart is 55, so your target zone is 83–123 beats per minute. Be aware that the figures in the table are averages, so use them as general guidelines.

A Note About Medications

A few high blood pressure medicines lower the maximum heart rate and thus the target zone rate. If you're taking high blood pressure medications, contact your doctor to report your target heart rate zone and to find out whether your activity program needs to be adjusted.

Taking Your Pulse

To find out whether you're within your target heart rate zone, take your pulse immediately after finishing your activity. Here's how:

- As soon as you stop your activity, place the tips of your first two fingers lightly over one of the two blood vessels on your neck, located to the left and right of your Adam's apple. Another convenient pulse spot is on the inside of your wrist, just below the base of your thumb.

- Count your pulse for 10 seconds and multiply by six.

- If your pulse falls within your target zone, your activity is providing good benefits for your heart and lungs. If you're below your target heart rate zone, move just a bit faster next time, as long as you continue to feel reasonably comfortable doing so. If you're above your target zone, move a little more slowly. Don't try to move at, or very close to, your maximum heart rate—that's working too hard.

- Eventually, you'll be consistently engaging in your activity within your target zone. To continue to track your progress, keep checking your pulse after at least one activity session per week.

A Sample Walking Program

During each week of the program, try to walk briskly at least 5 days per week. Always start with a 5 minute, slower paced walk to warm up, and end with a 5 minute, slower paced walk to cool down. (Warm up and cool down sessions totaling 10 minutes are included in the "total time" column.) As you walk, check your pulse periodically to see whether you're moving within your target heart rate zone.

Week	Warm up	Target zone	Cool down	Total time
Week 1	Walk 5 min.	Walk briskly 5 min.	Walk 5 min.	15 min.
Week 2	Walk 5 min.	Walk briskly 7 min.	Walk 5 min.	17 min.
Week 3	Walk 5 min.	Walk briskly 9 min.	Walk 5 min.	19 min.
Week 4	Walk 5 min.	Walk briskly 11 min.	Walk 5 min.	21 min.
Week 5	Walk 5 min.	Walk briskly 13 min.	Walk 5 min.	23 min.
Week 6	Walk 5 min.	Walk briskly 15 min.	Walk 5 min.	25 min.
Week 7	Walk 5 min.	Walk briskly 18 min.	Walk 5 min.	28 min.
Week 8	Walk 5 min.	Walk briskly 20 min.	Walk 5 min.	30 min.
Week 9	Walk 5 min.	Walk briskly 23 min.	Walk 5 min.	33 min.
Week 10	Walk 5 min.	Walk briskly 26 min.	Walk 5 min.	36 min.
Week 11	Walk 5 min.	Walk briskly 28 min.	Walk 5 min.	38 min.
Week 12	Walk 5 min.	Walk briskly 30 min.	Walk 5 min.	40 min.
Week 13 on:	Walk 5 min.	Continue. (See below.)	Walk 5 min.	

As you become more fit, try to walk within the upper range of your target zone. Gradually increase your brisk walking time from 30 to 60 minutes, most days of the week. Enjoy the outdoors!

A Sample Jogging Program

During each week of the program, try to jog at least 5 days per week. For your warm up, walk for 5 minutes. For your cool down, walk for 3 minutes and then stretch for 2 minutes more. (Warm up and cool down sessions totaling 10 minutes are included in the "total time" column.) As you jog, check your pulse periodically to see whether you're moving within your target heart rate zone. If you're over 40 and haven't been active in a while, begin with the walking program. After you complete the walking program, start with Week 3 of the jogging program.

Week	Warm up
Week 1	Walk 5 min., then stretch
Week 2	Walk 5 min., then stretch
Week 3	Walk 5 min., then stretch
Week 4	Walk 5 min., then stretch
Week 5	Walk 5 min., then stretch
Week 6	Walk 5 min., then stretch
Week 7	Walk 5 min., then stretch
Week 8	Walk 5 min., then stretch
Week 9	Walk 5 min., then stretch
Week 10	Walk 5 min., then stretch
Week 11	Walk 5 min., then stretch
Week 12	Walk 5 min., then stretch
Week 13	Walk 5 min., then stretch
Week 14	Walk 5 min., then stretch
Week 15	Walk 5 min., then stretch
Week 16 on:	Walk 5 min., then stretch

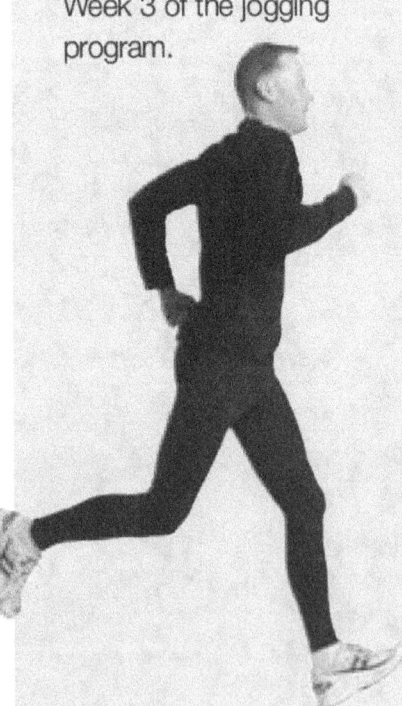

Jogging in your target zone	Cool down	Total time
Walk 10 min. Try to walk without stopping.	Walk 3 min., stretch 2 min.	20 min.
Walk 5 min., jog 1 min., walk 5 min., jog 1 min.	Walk 3 min., stretch 2 min.	22 min.
Walk 5 min., jog 3 min., walk 5 min., jog 3 min.	Walk 3 min., stretch 2 min.	26 min.
Walk 4 min., jog 5 min., walk 4 min., jog 5 min.	Walk 3 min., stretch 2 min.	28 min.
Walk 4 min., jog 5 min., walk 4 min., jog 5 min.	Walk 3 min., stretch 2 min.	28 min.
Walk 4 min., jog 6 min., walk 4 min., jog 6 min.	Walk 3 min., stretch 2 min.	30 min.
Walk 4 min., jog 7 min., walk 4 min., jog 7 min.	Walk 3 min., stretch 2 min.	32 min.
Walk 4 min., jog 8 min., walk 4 min., jog 8 min.	Walk 3 min., stretch 2 min.	34 min.
Walk 4 min., jog 9 min., walk 4 min., jog 9 min.	Walk 3 min., stretch 2 min.	36 min.
Walk 4 min., jog 13 min.	Walk 3 min., stretch 2 min.	27 min.
Walk 4 min., jog 15 min.	Walk 3 min., stretch 2 min.	29 min.
Walk 4 min., jog 17 min.	Walk 3 min., stretch 2 min.	31 min.
Walk 2 min., jog slowly 2 min., jog 17 min.	Walk 3 min., stretch 2 min.	31 min.
Walk 1 min., jog slowly 3 min., jog 17 min.	Walk 3 min., stretch 2 min.	31 min.
Jog slowly 3 min., jog 17 min.	Walk 3 min., stretch 2 min.	30 min.
Continue. (See below.)	Walk 3 min., stretch 2 min.	

As you become more fit, try to jog within the upper range of your target zone. Gradually, increase your jogging time from 20 to 30 minutes (or up to 60 minutes, if you wish). Keep track of your goals   and keep on enjoying yourself.

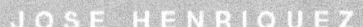

JOSE HENRIQUEZ

"I was overweight. I was told by my doctor that if I kept it up I was going to develop high blood pressure and high blood cholesterol. Once I realized no one was going to take care of me except me, I started eating better and exercising. I go to a gym every day from Monday through Friday. I take a spinning class, I do weight lifting, and I use the machines. I feel younger when I go to the gym, like I can do anything. When I don't go to the gym I can tell the difference—my stamina is gone."

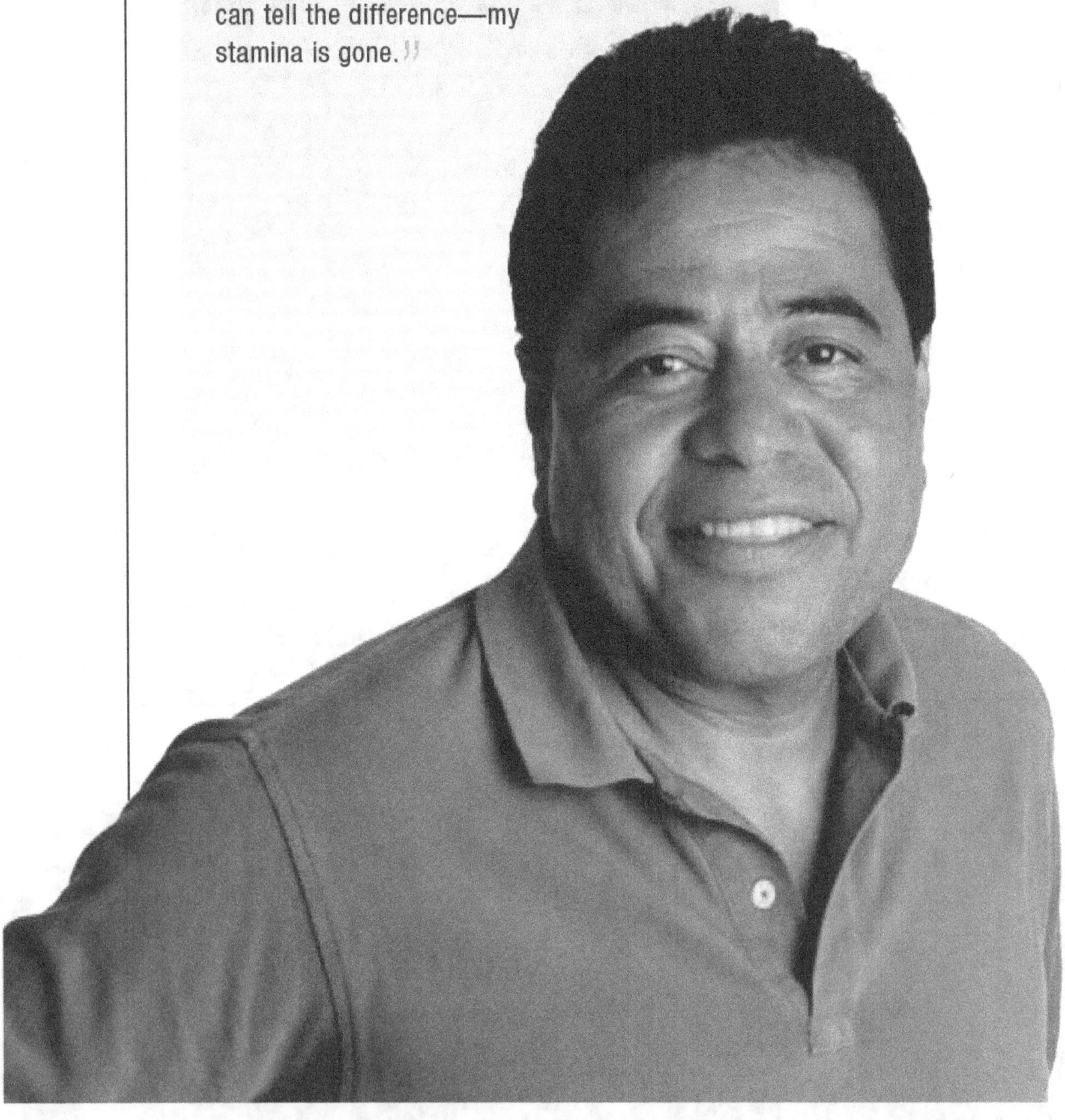

Playing It Safe

By and large, physical activity is a very safe way to help protect your heart. But like anything else you do, getting fit requires taking a few common-sense precautions. Following are some important safety tips:

Avoid Injury

- It can't be said too often: Start your activity program gradually, and work up slowly. Be sure to warm up, cool down, and stretch each and every time you are physically active. Exercising too much, too fast, can cause injuries.

- A certain amount of stiffness is normal at first. But if you do hurt a joint or pull a muscle, stop the activity for several days to avoid more serious injury. Rest and over-the-counter painkillers can heal most minor muscle and joint problems.

- Use proper equipment. Wear good shoes with adequate cushioning in the soles for jogging or walking. Use goggles to protect your eyes for sports such as handball or racquetball.

- Joggers should run on soft, even surfaces such as a level grass field, a dirt path, or a track. Hard or uneven surfaces, such as cement or rough fields, are more likely to cause injuries. Also, try to land on your heels, rather than on the balls of your feet, to minimize strain on your feet and lower legs.

- If you jog or walk on the street, watch for cars. Wear light-colored clothing with a reflecting band at night so that drivers can see you more easily. Always face oncoming traffic. Remember, drivers can't see you as well as you can see their cars.

- If you bicycle, always wear a helmet. Ride in the direction of traffic and try to avoid busy streets. At night, use lights and wheel-mounted reflectors.

Eat Right

- If you've just eaten a meal, avoid strenuous physical activity for at least 2 hours.

- If you've just been vigorously active, wait about 20 minutes before eating.

- If you plan to be continuously active for more than 60 minutes, you may want to take a snack along to keep up your energy level. Good choices are light foods and drinks that are high in carbohydrates, such as bananas, raisins, bagels, or sport drinks.

Check the Weather Report

On hot, humid days:
- Try to be physically active during the cooler and less humid parts of the day, such as early morning or early evening.

- Wear light, loose-fitting, "breathable" clothing. Never wear rubberized or plastic suits. Such clothing won't help you lose weight by making you sweat more, but it can cause dangerously high body temperatures.

- Drink adequate fluids—particularly water—before, during, and after your physical activity.

- Watch for symptoms of heat exhaustion and heat stroke. (See the box on page 33, "Taking Too Much Heat.")

On cold days:
- When dressing for outdoor activity, wear one layer less than you'd wear if you were outside but not physically active. Ideally wear several layers of clothing rather than one heavy jacket, so you can remove a layer if you get too warm.

- Use mittens, gloves, or cotton socks to protect your hands.

- Wear a hat, since up to 40 percent of your body heat is lost through your head and neck.

Taking Too Much Heat

When you're active outdoors in hot, humid weather, be alert for signs of heat exhaustion and heat stroke. Although many of their symptoms are similar, heat stroke is the more serious condition. Heat stroke occurs when the body temperature increases too much, causing stress on the body that may harm tissues. The rise in temperature occurs when the heat produced during exercise exceeds the heat that leaves the body. The following are the main symptoms of each type of heat problem:

Heat Exhaustion	Heat Stroke
Dizziness	Dizziness
Headache	Headache
Nausea	Nausea
Confusion	Confusion
Body temperature below normal	Muscle cramps
	Sweating stops
	High body temperature

Both heat exhaustion and heat stroke can be avoided by drinking enough water to replace fluids lost during physical activity. Drink water regularly throughout your activity, but don't "over water" yourself. Drink no more than 3 cups of water per hour.

On rainy, icy, or snowy days:

- Be aware of reduced visibility—for both yourself and for drivers—and reduced traction on roadways.

Seek Company

- If you're concerned about the safety of your surroundings, pair up with a buddy for outdoor activities. If possible, walk, bike, or jog during daylight hours.

- Check out the hours of nearby shopping malls. Many malls are open early and late for people who prefer to walk or jog at those times of day, but in a safe, well-lit area. (Indoor malls also make it possible to stay active during summer heat, winter cold, and allergy seasons.)

Know the Signs of a Heart Problem

While physical activity can strengthen your heart, some types of activity may worsen existing heart problems. Warning signals include sudden dizziness, cold sweat, paleness, fainting, extreme breathlessness, or pain or pressure in your upper body. These symptoms may occur during, or just after, an activity. Ignoring these signals and continuing your activity may lead to serious heart problems. Instead, call your doctor right away.

Get Back in the Swing

If you have to miss a few sessions of physical activity because of illness or injury, don't be discouraged. Once you recover, you can get right back on the "activity track." But *do* wait until you recover. If you come down with a minor illness, such as a cold, wait until you feel normal before you resume your activity. If you suffer a minor injury, wait until the pain disappears before continuing. When you do resume your fitness sessions, start at one-half to two-thirds of your previous level, depending on the number of days you've missed and how you feel while moving.

If your activity program has been interrupted by a major illness or injury, consult your doctor about the best time—and pace—for resuming your fitness program. Whatever your reasons for missing sessions, don't worry about the skipped days or weeks. Just get back into your routine and focus on the progress you'll be making toward your fitness goals.

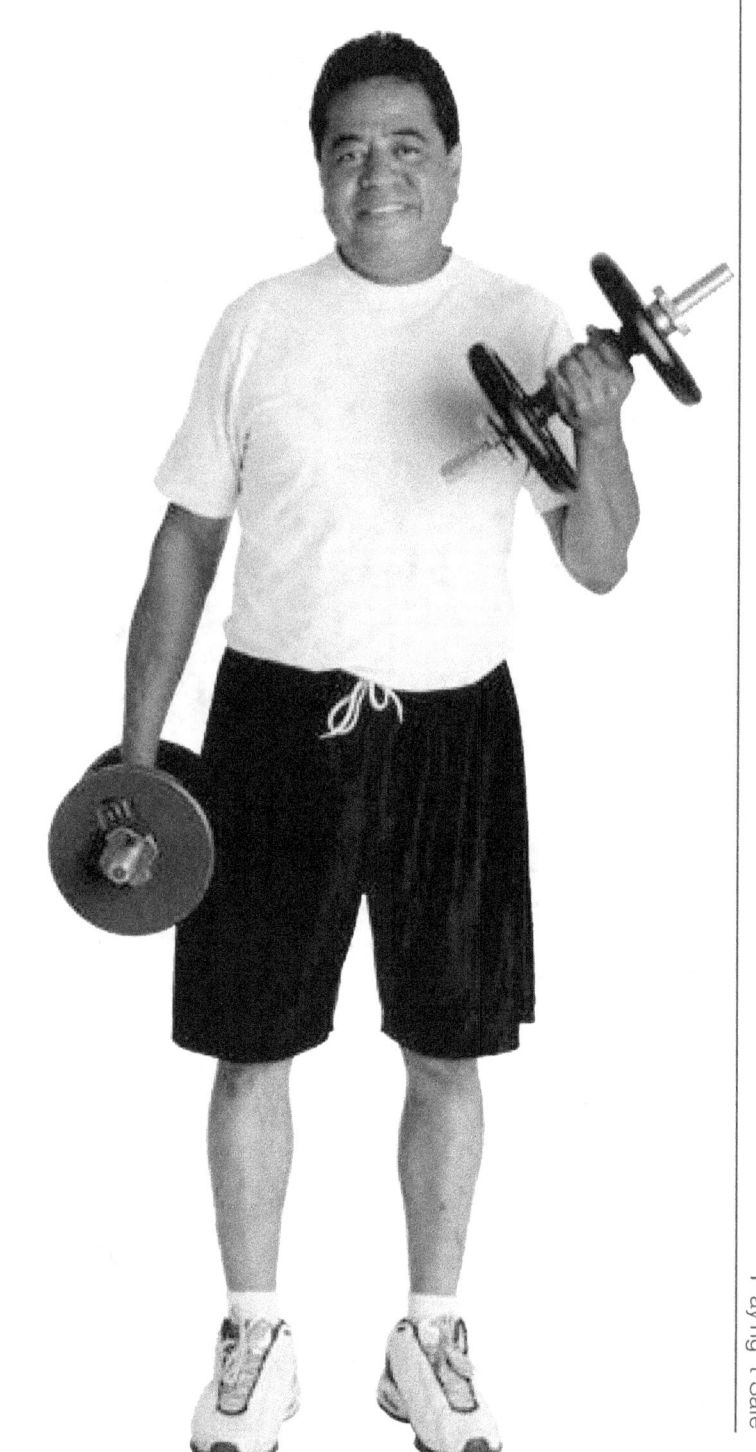

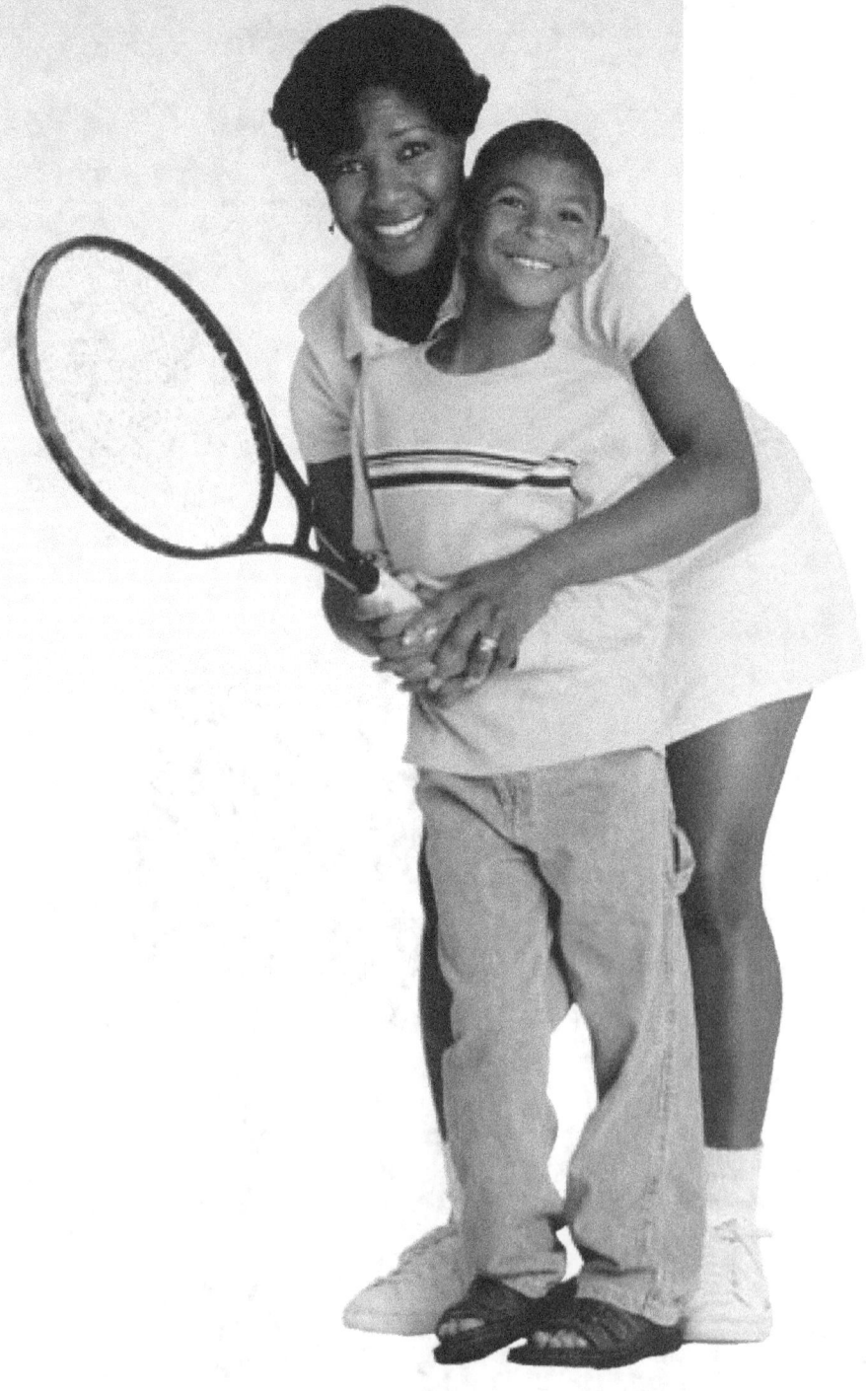

JEANETTE GUYTON-KRISHNAN
AND IAN

"We exercise regularly, not as much as
we should, but we do try. We have a treadmill
and weights at home. My son is active in
tennis, baseball, and soccer."

Staying Active

Becoming physically active is the first step in a heart healthy fitness plan. Now comes the more challenging part—*staying* active. After a while, it may be tempting to put off that regular walk or bike ride, especially when you get busy or the weather doesn't cooperate. Yet, to keep your heart healthy, and to keep your body strong and fit overall, staying physically active over time is very important. Here are some tips for making physical activity an enjoyable, habitual part of your life.

Motivation Makers

- **Think short-term as well as long-term.** If your long-term goal is to walk 1 mile, then make your short-term goal much smaller. How about walking a quarter mile during the first week? Similarly, if one of your long-term goals is to lose 15 pounds, focus first on a more immediate, "doable" goal. How about losing 1–2 pounds the first week? You get the idea. By setting smaller goals within your bigger ones, you're less likely to push yourself too hard. Just as important, you give yourself a chance to succeed—over and over.

- **Share your activity goals with others.** Encouragement from family and friends can help motivate you to stay active. Let others know your short-term goals as well as your long-term ones, so they can regularly cheer you on. And who knows, you may be able to persuade family or friends to join in! (For ideas on getting family members involved, see the box, "Family Fitness," on page 39.)

- **Help yourself remember.** You may want to stay active but sometimes forget your fitness sessions because, well, life gets busy. Leave your sneakers near the door to remind yourself to walk, or bring a change of clothes to work and head straight for the gym, yoga class, or walking trail on the way home. Make a "personal activity checklist" and stick it on the fridge or another spot where you'll see it daily.

■ **Recall your original reasons for getting fit.** Why did you decide to start your activity program in the first place? Do these reasons still apply, or are others now more important? Taking a look at your original goals and desires can help to rev up your motivation, or allow you to pinpoint where to make changes. If you find that you're no longer enjoying a particular activity, consider trying out a new one.

Creating Opportunities

It's easier to stay physically active over time if you take advantage of everyday opportunities to move around. For example:

■ Use the stairs—both up and down—instead of the elevator. Start with one flight of stairs and gradually build up to more.

■ Park a few blocks from the office or store and walk the rest of the way. If you take public transportation, get off a stop or two early and walk a few blocks.

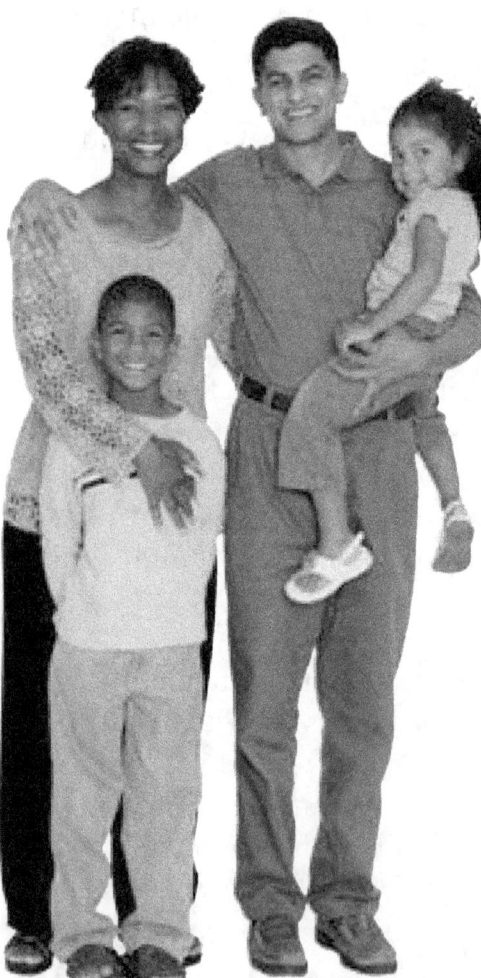

■ While working, take frequent activity breaks. Get up and stretch, walk around, and give your muscles and mind a chance to relax.

■ Instead of eating that extra snack, take a brisk stroll around the neighborhood or your office building.

■ Do housework, gardening, or yard work at a more vigorous pace.

■ When you travel, walk around the train station, bus station, or airport rather than sitting and waiting.

Family Fitness

When it comes to getting in shape, what's good for you is good for your whole family. Children and teenagers should be physically active for at least 60 minutes per day. A great way to pry kids off the couch — and help *you* to stay fit as well — is to do enjoyable activities together. Some ideas:

- **Kick up your heels.** Take turns picking out your favorite music and dance up a storm in the living room.
- **Explore the outdoors.** Hit your local trail on weekends for some biking or hiking. Pack a healthy lunch and let the kids choose the picnic spot.
- **Get classy.** Join family members in an active class, such as martial arts, yoga, or aerobics.
- **Play pupil.** Ask one of your children or grandchildren to teach you an active game or sport. Kids love to be the experts — and you'll get a workout learning a new activity!
- **Use online resources.** Check out the "**We Can!**" Web site at http://wecan.nhlbi.nih.gov There you'll find more family friendly ideas for making smart food choices, increasing physical activity, and reducing "screen time" in front of the TV and other electronic attractions.

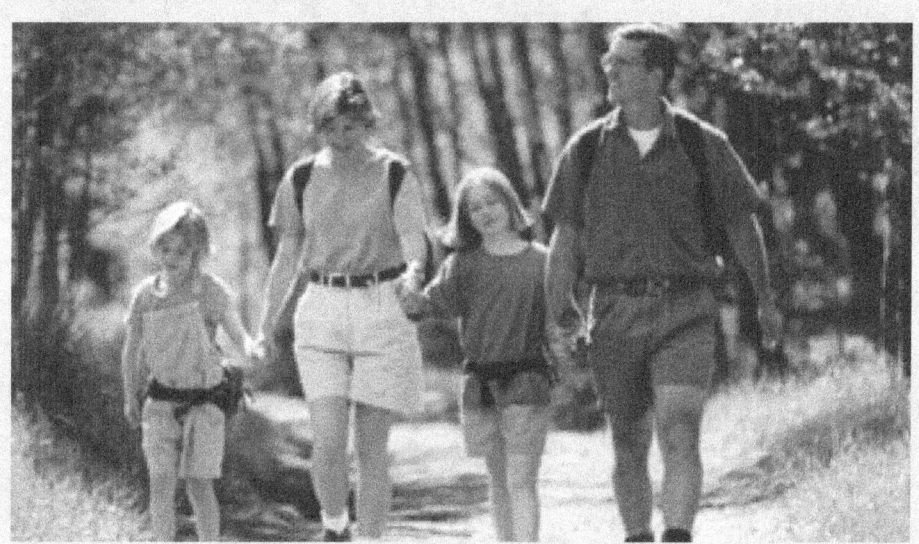

■ Keep moving while you watch TV. Lift hand weights, do some gentle yoga stretches, or pedal an exercise bike.

■ Better yet, turn off the TV and take a brisk walk.

You may be pleasantly surprised at how many miles you log in a day or week, just by taking advantage of everyday opportunities. To keep track, consider using a pedometer. (See the box below, "Measuring Your Mileage.")

Measuring Your Mileage

Using a pedometer is an excellent way to motivate yourself to stay physically active. A pedometer is a small counting device that measures the number of steps you walk. Just clip the device to your waistband and watch your steps add up. You can set goals for the number of steps you take every day and challenge yourself to take more steps each week.

One mile equals roughly 2,000 steps, or 15 minutes of physical activity. Physical activities that don't involve steps, such as weight lifting or swimming, will not register on your pedometer. But they still count, of course, toward your daily physical activity goal.

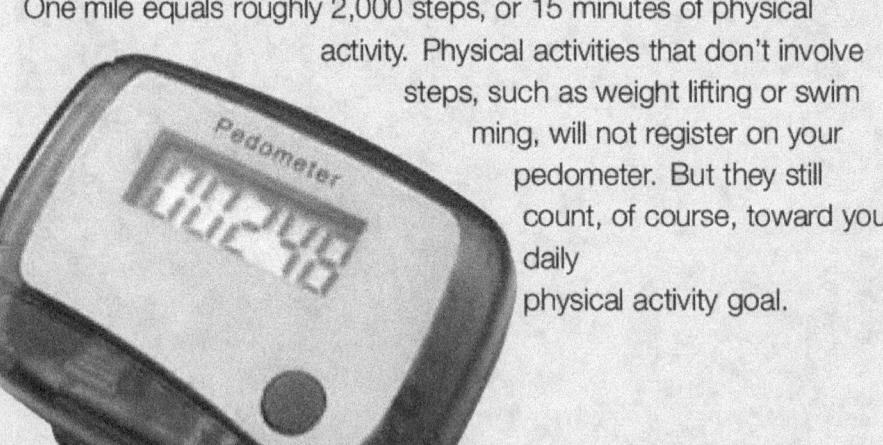

Moving Toward Health

Becoming physically active may start as a reminder note on your calendar and then become—when you least expect it—a habit and a pleasure. As you strengthen your heart, you may find that getting fit also gives you more energy, stamina, and ability to cope with the ups and downs of daily life. The fact is, getting regular physical activity is one of the single best choices you can make for yourself and your health.

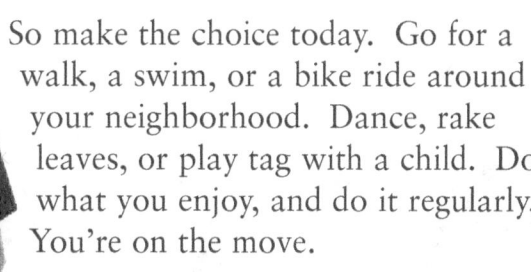

So make the choice today. Go for a walk, a swim, or a bike ride around your neighborhood. Dance, rake leaves, or play tag with a child. Do what you enjoy, and do it regularly. You're on the move.

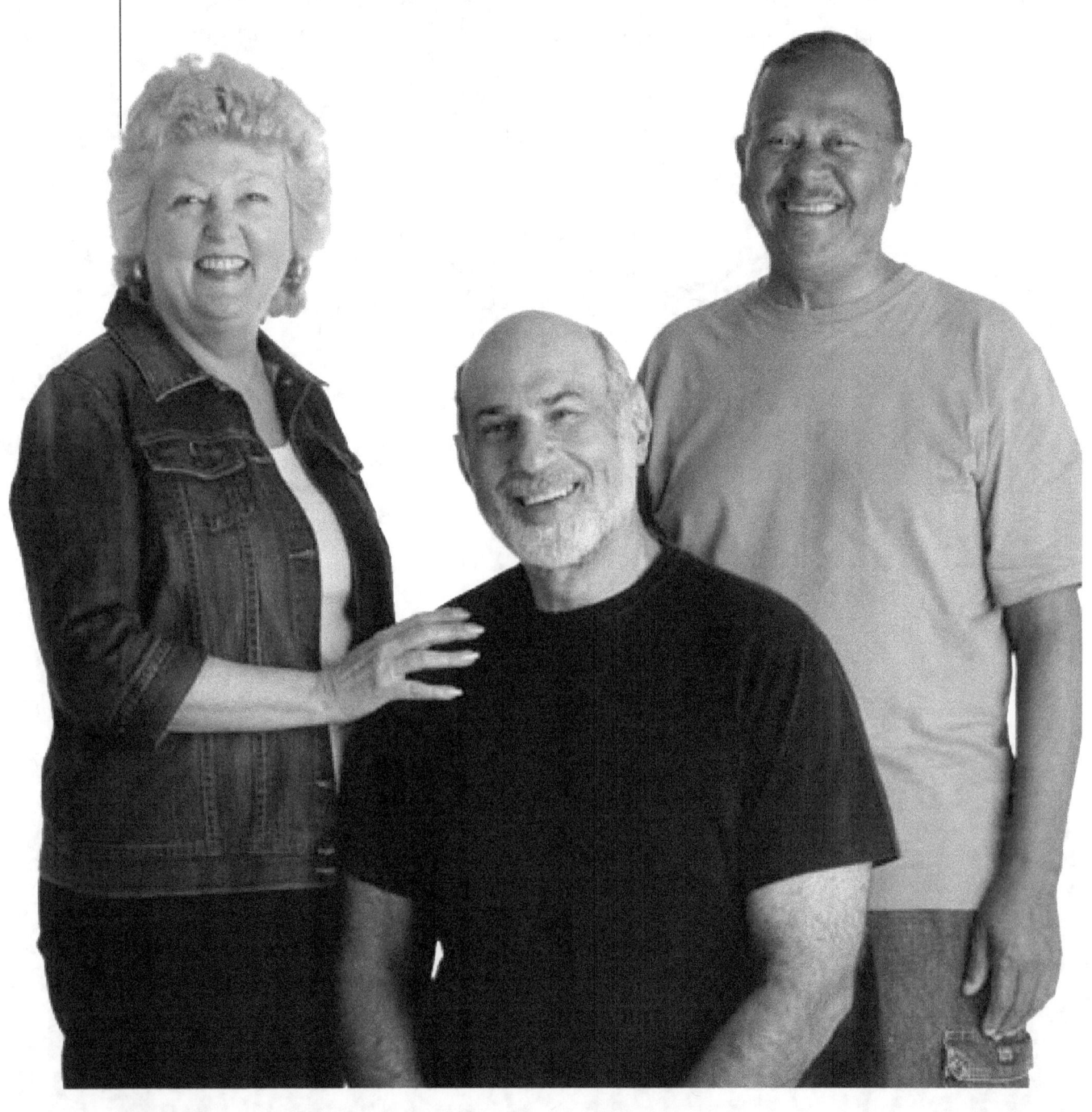

To Learn More

The National Heart, Lung, and Blood Institute (NHLBI) provides information on the prevention and treatment of heart disease and offers publications on heart health and heart disease.

NHLBI Health Information Center
P.O. Box 30105
Bethesda, MD 20824-0105
Phone: 301–592–8573
TTY: 240–629–3255
Fax: 301–592–8563

NHLBI Heart Health Information Line
1–800–575–WELL
Provides toll-free recorded messages.

Also, check out these NHLBI Web sites and Web pages:

NHLBI Web site: www.nhlbi.nih.gov

Diseases and Conditions A–Z Index:
   www.nhlbi.nih.gov/health/dci/index.html

Aim for a Healthy Weight:
   http://healthyweight.nhlbi.nih.gov

The Heart Truth: A National Awareness Campaign for Women About
   Heart Disease: www.hearttruth.com

Your Guide to Lowering High Blood Pressure:
   www.nhlbi.nih.gov/hbp/index.html

Live Healthier, Live Longer (on lowering elevated blood cholesterol):
   www.nhlbi.nih.gov/chd

We Can! (Ways to Enhance Children's Activity and Nutrition): http://wecan.nhlbi.nih.gov or call toll-free at 1–866–35WECAN

Other Web sites and Web pages on physical activity:

American College of Sports Medicine: www.acsm.org/health%2Bfitness/index.htm

President's Council on Physical Fitness: www.fitness.gov

Exercising Safely for Seniors: www.nihseniorhealth.org/exercise/toc.html

For more information on heart health, see MedlinePlus: www.medlineplus.gov